HELP

WITH YOUR PROJECT

A guide for students of health care

Dianne Owen and
Moya Davis

Edward Arnold
A member of the Hodder Headline Group
LONDON   MELBOURNE   AUCKLAND

9203058

WX 20

2nd copy.

First published in Great Britain 1991 by
Edward Arnold, a division of Hodder Headline PLC,
338 Euston Road, London NW1 3BH

British Library Cataloguing in Publication Data
Owen, Dianne
Help with your project: A guide to students of health care.
I. Title II. Davis, Moya
362.1071

ISBN 0-340-55270-0

3 4 5 6 7   94 95 96 97 98

Typeset in Goudy Old Style by The Design Team, Ascot
Printed and bound in Great Britain by
Ashford Overload, Southampton

Contents

Acknowledgements

The authors gratefully acknowledge the advice and help given by Roger Davis, MBE, during the development of this guide.

1
Using this Guide

Introduction

This guide has been prepared to help you, as a student of health care whether at pre or post qualification level, to plan, carry out and present a simple research project. This type of project may be required as part of a management or other type of course, or as a part of everyday work. Such projects often differ from the majority of academic work submitted to others for their opinion, in that you, the researcher, may not have an academic adviser at your elbow to guide you through the various stages. This guide aims to overcome the problem of the absent tutor by providing you with 'tutors in text', Dianne Owen, a professional researcher, and Moya Davis, a lecturer. They have worked closely with many health care professionals who have had to undertake small projects as part of their work or of courses which they are attending. In preparing this guide the authors have drawn on their experience of the questions they have been asked, and the help and advice that has been given.

The Chapters

The guide has been prepared in nine chapters. The first four chapters consider your study strategy and general research groundwork and methods, so that you have a good basis from which to develop your project. Without this information you may waste a lot of time on unsound research and have to retrace your steps at a later stage. The last five chapters then guide you through the stages of your own project. The individual chapters are as follows:

This first chapter describes how the method of study works and helps you to get the maximum benefit from it.

Chapter 2   Project? What project?   looks at the variety of reasons for undertaking simple research and helps you to identify your own project time scale.

Chapter 3   What type of project?   examines different types of research project and helps you to consider their relevance to your own area of health care.

Chapter 4   Methods of investigation   considers the ways in which research information can be collected, again applying them to your own possible research needs.

Chapter 5   Your project proposal   helps you to put together the proposal for the research which you are to undertake,

Chapter 6   Searching the literature   takes you through the process of finding out what has been written or recorded on the subject by other people, thus saving you reinventing the wheel.

Chapter 7   Obtaining your own data   helps you to develop methods of obtaining and recording the information you require.

Chapter 8   Analysing your data   describes various methods of analysis and graphic presentation of findings.

Chapter 9   Reporting your results   draws your work to its conclusion with the writing and submission and 'live' presentation of your project report.

At the beginning of each chapter you will find a short **check list** of the ground you should expect to have covered by the time you have completed that chapter.

As you work through the text of each chapter you will encounter a number of **action boxes, describing tasks** which you should complete as you meet them, These boxes are an important part of the guide because they enable you to immediately apply information, given in the text, to your own project. Provide yourself with a notebook or loose leaf file in which to enter the completed tasks so that they build up into a personal 'project resource'. At the end of each chapter there is a short **summary** to help you recap on the ground covered. In the **reference and further reading** sections you will find a list of books which we think may be useful if you require additional information on any aspect of your project.

Study Aim

The overall aim for study of this guide is that when you have worked through it you will have:

Completed a simple research project to your own satisfaction and to that of those requiring you to undertake it.

We hope that you will find the guide helpful.

2
Project? What Project?

Check list

When you have completed this chapter you should have:

● Identified your reasons for undertaking a research project

● Set intended and absolute completion dates

● Established a workable weekly time allocation for the project

Why do a Project?

All right, let's get 'because somebody told me to' out of the way right now! You have our sympathy but there still has to be a reason why someone wants you to put in all this effort.

The reasons for carrying out the project will have a great deal of influence on many factors which will contribute to the end result, how much time you have available between now and the project completion date, if there is one, for a start! We have no way of knowing your own individual reason but some of the most common are:

● In response to a request at work. This could be as part of a working party or planning review group. In some cases such groups feel that they lack information, and allocate research to one or more members. Alternatively, it could be a request from a line manager.

● In response to a problem which you have identified during your work and which you think requires investigation.

● As part of a course of study. This situation is different from the others in that you are not acting in response to a problem, you have to think one up!

● Identifying a research project can sometimes be difficult but your colleagues or managers may have some helpful ideas.

Identify your reasons for undertaking a research project by completing your first Action Box. Note down the instructions in the box, as well as your response, in your file. In this way you will not look back at your file and wonder what each of your notes refers to!

ACTION BOX 2.1

Identify the reason/s why you are undertaking a project.

Time Constraints

The next factor which you need to think through with some care is the amount of time which you have available. Some authors may be able to reel off a best seller in a few weeks but less lucky individuals cannot count on such a free flow of the pen. Besides, your project will involve research, meticulously planned, carried out and evaluated, in comparison with which dashing off a best seller might be a doddle. So, do you have a submission deadline which you must meet for this project, or can you set your own? That gives a fair range between 'tomorrow at noon' and 'when the new intake are drawing their pensions'. Most people have a completion date imposed on them, with no bargaining. Identify your completion date and vow that you will stick to it. Having identified the actual completion date, set a second target date within it by taking off at least one week for a three month project, two weeks for a six month project, and one month for a twelve

---

ACTION BOX 2.2

Note down your unavoidable and absolutely not negotiable completion date. Next, work out your intended earlier completion date, for which you will now aim.

month project. In this way you will build in some 'unforeseen slippage' time which, although termed 'unforeseen', almost always occurs.

Next, how many hours per week are you going to be able to devote to the project? Is it to be carried out in work time or, for example if it is part of an external course of study, in your own time?

ACTION BOX 2.3

Have a look at your own situation now and set a realistic weekly time allocation for your project work. Identify your strategy, such as using two afternoons of work time, or your own time in the mornings of your late shifts, and so on. You may find the steps below helpful in doing this.

		Tick
My project work will be carried out	- in my own time	☐
	- in work time	☐
	- some of each	☐
I hope to allocate the following hours	- up to 5 per week	☐
	- 6 to 10 per week	☐
	- 11 to 15 per week	☐
	- over 15 per week	☐

I will achieve this by setting aside the following times for project work:

You have identified your strategy, now stick to it!

Chapter summary
In this chapter we have discussed different reasons for undertaking a research project. We have advised on the sense of setting early target, and final completion, dates and the identification of a weekly time allocation for project work.

3
What Type of Project?

Check list

When you have completed this chapter you should have:

● Considered three main categories of research project

● Identified at least one example of each category from your own work area

Perhaps it seems odd to have looked at time constraints before considering the type of project on which you may embark. However, it is no good identifying 'the five year development programme' of your health district or organisation if your project submission date is Friday week. Keep your time constraints in mind as we discuss the different types of project which you may consider. If you have already identified a subject for your project, or had one identified for you, we think you will find it helpful to work through this chapter all the same, because we hope that it will increase your overall understanding of research.

Projects can usefully be divided into three broad categories according to their purpose:

● to investigate and review an existing system or practice

● to evaluate the effect of changes which have already taken place

● to look at the possibilities for introducing new systems or practices

Have a look at each of them now, and for each type identify a suitable subject in your own work area by completing the next three exercises as you come to them.

Investigation and Review

Such a review examines an existing system or practice and can lead to recommendations for change. An example of this could be the streamlining of paperwork and administrative systems. If you have ever wondered 'Why on earth do we fill in Forms A, B, and C?' this type of project might suit you. Equally, a review of training provision, both in your health care organisation and in others, could lead to the rationalisation of input or the development of new ideas. Some clinical research projects also come into this category, for example evaluating the effectiveness of a treatment or method of care that has been used for a considerable period. We may continue to use the same techniques because we think from everyday observation that they work, without evaluating accurately how effective they really are. Our everyday impressions may be right, but they may equally well be wrong!

ACTION BOX 3.1

Consider whether an 'investigation and review' project could be undertaken in your work area and list two or three possible subjects. This does not mean that you are committing yourself to this type of research at this stage, just opening up your mind to the possibilities.

Evaluation of Change

Change is always with us, sometimes forced upon us. It is easy and very tempting to make off the cuff evaluations of the effects of change, but such evaluations have no credibility and serve no purpose except, perhaps, to let off steam. Structured evaluation, on the other hand, can give irrefutable answers that can be used to support, or bring about revision of, the change.

A type of research termed **action research falls into this category**. It considers a problem in a specific context and attempts to solve it in that context, with team members themselves taking part in implementing the research. Changes are continuously evaluated with the aim of improving practice in some way or other (Cohen and Manion 1989).

Examples of subjects for this type of evaluation are changes in staffing levels in a community area, ward or department leading to alterations in standards of care. Another example is patient/client satisfaction level resulting from changes, however small, in management of such items as admission procedures. How could this type of evaluation fit into the needs of your work area? Clinical research often comes into this category encompassing items such as the effectiveness of changes in drug regimes or the effect of an an innovative dietary supplement on the progress of people with a particular medical condition. Be warned that these types of project are very involved and complex because there are so many other factors that could effect how well people receiving the treatment may do. Clinical research generally is more difficult to set up, monitor and evaluate than that into non-clinical areas of health care. Additionally, clinical research has potentially greater ethical problems than other types of research. We shall consider obtaining advice on ethical aspects of your project in Chapter 5.

ACTION BOX 3.2

List two or three subjects that an 'evaluation of change' project in your work area could examine.

New Systems or Practices

This type of project fills a void by formulating a system or practice where none has existed before. An example of this could be a staff or peer group appraisal system. Alternatively, do you have a system for allocating holidays rather than the 'Bloggins Books First' lottery with which most of us are familiar? What about a system for monitoring waiting times in radiography, haematology or other specialist departments?

ACTION BOX 3.3

Have a look at the organisation of your own work area and see if you can identify any 'system or practice' voids which you think could do with filling. List two or three items for which you have no existing system.

That completes the work of this chapter.

Chapter summary

In this chapter we have looked at three main categories of research projects, investigation and review, evaluation of change and new system or practice formulation.

Reference

Cohen C. and Manion L. (1989). *Research methods in education* 3rd Edition. Routledge, London.

4
Methods of Investigation

Check list

When you have completed this chapter you should have:

● Become aware of the limitations of published statistics

● Obtained information on data already collected within your organisation

● Identified useful subjects for collection of data by observation or self
recording

● Gained an understanding of two ways of conducting a survey

Having examined different categories of research projects we can now look at the
different ways in which reliable data can be obtained. By data we mean 'facts that
have been gathered'. We are still talking generally here. We shall start to get to
grips with your actual project in the next chapter.

Finding Information

Before you begin any investigative project you need to specify all the different
types of information you will require. You will also need to identify the sources
from which you hope to obtain the information and the order in which you will
require it

Since time constraints are usually a major factor, a systematic approach to planning your collection of data can save you a great deal of effort. Remember that after you have collected the information you will have to spend time analysing it and in writing your report, so you will need to keep your completion date in mind. The 'before slippage' one, that is!

There are four common sources of information which you should consider either individually or in combination when designing your project:

- abstraction from published statistics

- data already collected within your organisation or field of study

- observation and self recording

- surveys

Have a look at each of them now in some detail.

Published Statistics

There is a wide variety of published statistical information readily available including:

Government statistics
Each government department produces its own statistics which are published through Her Majesty's Stationery Office (HMSO).

Two useful and readily available guides to these statistics are:

'*Government statistics — a brief guide to sources*'. This will be kept in most reference libraries and is also available from:

Information Services Division,
Cabinet Office,
Great George Street,
London. SWIP 3AL.

The booklet lists publications and also gives a summary under broad headings of those which might be useful for different subject areas. In addition to being available in libraries, government statistics publications may be purchased from booksellers who are HMSO stockists.

'*Central Statistical Office — Guide to Official Statistics*. This is revised at intervals and an up-to-date edition will be kept in most reference libraries. It is a much more detailed publication than the brief guide mentioned above. It aims to give the user an indication of whether the statistics required have been compiled and if so where they have been published. The publication covers all official statistics but some examples for areas relevant to health care are given below. Several references are given in the guide for each of the following headings.

Vital statistics

a. Publications of the Office of Population Censuses and Surveys
b. Publications of the Registrars General for Scotland and Northern Ireland
c. Births
d. Fertility rates and mean family size
e. Marriages and divorces
f. Deaths
g. Deaths by cause
h. Infant and meternal mortality
i. Life tables and expectation of life
j. British vital statistics compared with those of other countries
k. Family planning

National Health Service: General Statistics

a. Notifications of infectious diseases
b. Sexually transmitted diseases
c. Cancer, cervical cytology
d. Abortions
e. Congenital malformations
f. Incidence of sickness
g. Smoking and drinking
h. National Health Service finance
i. National Health Service statistics, general manpower: medical education

The Hospital Services

a. Finance of the hospital services
b. Hospital staffs
c. General hospital statistics (number of hospitals, beds, patients etc.)
d. Inpatient statistics
e. Specialist services (e.g. blood transfusions, mass radiography)

Other National Health Services

a.   General medical practitioner services
b.   Pharmaceutical services
c.   General dental services
d.   General ophthalmic services
e.   Community health services
f.   School health service
g.   Other services (e.g. ambulances)

Two useful annual publications produced by HMSO which are referenced many times in the Official Statistics Guide are:

Social trends. Includes national statistics on population, education, employment, income, expenditure, health, housing, transport and law enforcement.

Regional trends. Contains the same types of information as 'Social trends' but by region.

Other statistics

CIPFA statistics. The Chartered Institute of Public Finance and Accountancy produces a range of local government statistics. These include demographic and workload figures in addition to financial information, and allow comparisons to be made between relevant areas e.g. counties, police forces and so on. Any comparisons made must be treated with caution as each area fills in its own return and there could be multiple interpretations of the same instructions.

Annual reports and statistics. This covers not only company reports, which include financial accounts, but also those of universities, police forces, councils, health authorities and other publicly funded bodies. It also includes charities and voluntary organisations. Some may have to be obtained by writing to the organisation itself.

The above list is just for 'starters'! Other useful places through which statistics may be traced are quality newspapers, magazines and professional journals. You will need to follow up such leads by obtaining the original report from which the paper obtained its information.

Interpretation of Statistics

It is essential to investigate the accuracy of data from all published sources as there may have been errors of interpretation or transcription.

It is therefore important, when you are using such information, to understand the basis on which it has been compiled, and you should always make a critical analysis of who requested, and who carried out, the collection of the data. You should also examine the method of presentation of the data to consider whether it gives a more favourable view than might otherwise be so, given the use to which the data has been put. The example we give here shows how doing something simple such as altering the scale on a graph can distort the information being presented.

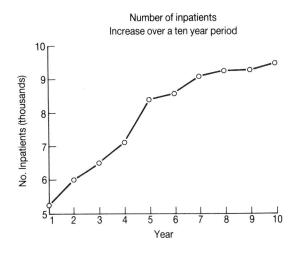

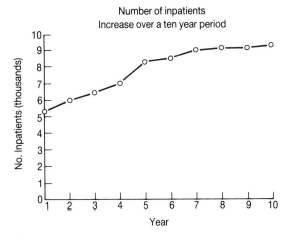

These graphs contain the same figures, the only difference is the vertical scale used. The graph on the left with a scale starting at 5 gives the impression that inpatient numbers have increased dramatically over the 10 year period. The graph on the right with the scale starting at 0 gives the impression of a much more gradual rise.

Now have a look at the statement and graph which follow and see if you can spot any flaws in the argument, then complete the Action Box.

'The increase in visits per district nurse from year 1 to year 2 was greatest in area C, therefore some district nurses should be transfered from A and B to C.'

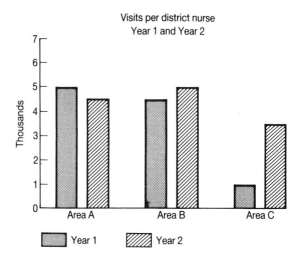

After this particular Action Box we shall discuss possible answers, but please do have a go at spotting the errors yourself. Part of the reason for completing this chapter is to increase your own ability to evaluate these problems in the future.

ACTION BOX 4.1

Describe the flaws in the argument as you see them.

Some possible comments that you may have made are:

● Visits per district nurse have risen more in area C but are still lower in year 2 than in areas A and B.

● We do not know the cause of the increase in the area C ratio, it could have been due to an increase in visits, a decrease in nurses or a combination of both. Is this change likely to be temporary or permanent? How were the variables used in calculating the ratio, i.e. number of visits and number of nurses, defined? For example, was the nurse figure based on actual days worked during the year or the establishment number of nurses?

● Some types of patient will require longer visits than others and the three areas could have different patient mixes. There could be large differences in the number of visits made but only small differences in the amount of time spent visiting.

● The number of visits that could be made would vary according to geographic factors. For example if area C is very rural whereas A and B are urban you would expect nurses in area C to have to spend a higher proportion of their time travelling and a lower proportion with patients.

Remember to look at published information critically and bear the possibility of such distortions, whether intentional or not, in mind.

Data Already Collected

If you are evaluating an existing system it will be necessary to obtain all the relevant information currently collected. Where this can be obtained from will obviously depend on the subject of your investigation. In some cases, such as the number of outpatients attending a clinic, the information may be readily available. In others, such as the number of cases where outpatients with appointments did not attend, the information may be less easy to obtain. You may have to sort through past clinic lists and count nonattenders.
    Now complete Action Box 4.2 (overleaf).

These last two sections have considered existing sources of information. The next two sections cover situations where you have to collect data yourself.

Observation and Self Recording

If a researcher observes the actions of a group without being a member of it the observation is termed **nonparticipant**. In this way you might, as a medical social worker concerned about the difficulties of patients discussing their fears with medical staff, observe a series of interviews between patients and doctors. Another example is observing how long a ward sister spends on the telephone each day.
    Where a researcher takes part in the activities that are being observed, as a member of the group, the observation is known as **participant observation**

ACTION BOX 4.2

Think of an existing system in your work area on which data is already collected and then complete the details below:

Investigation of an existing system could be as follows:

System:

Possible investigation:

Data required:

Method by which it could be obtained, including persons doing the recording:

(Cohen and Manion 1989). This type of observation may be useful if, for example, you wish to review evidence of attitudes of the group of which you are a member in particular aspects of care, such as communication with relatives of dying patients. If the researcher tells the group that the observations are to be made, and obtains their agreement, the research is made openly and is termed **overt**. If the group are not told that their behaviour is to be observed and recorded the resulting undercover research is termed **covert**. Covert participant observation can be held to have great ethical implications. Can you, as a health care professional, ethically justify observing the behaviour of your colleagues without telling them what you are doing? Covert observation of clients is even more problematic and we shall discuss its implications in Chapter 5.

In a relatively small and simple research project the drawbacks of observation and self recording are considerable. In addition to the potential ethical problems they are very time consuming methods and will not be suitable in many cases. The difference between them in practical terms is that observation uses your own time and self recording uses the time of the people doing the job. Two examples where these methods might be useful are:

● **timing** – for example how long it takes to enter one piece of information into a computer. This may indicate that operators are as overworked as they have been saying! Another example is how long community midwives spend on travelling and administration. They could be asked to keep a diary of everything they do, with times, for a specified number of days. This is a useful approach if you want to find out what type of work people do and what proportion of their time they spend on different activities.

● **counting** – for example the number of requests for different information made by patients in a hospital ward. This sort of information could lead to the production of new information leaflets.

Identify an item in your work or study area where observation or self recording would be an appropriate and useful method of collecting data.

ACTION BOX 4.3

Identify an item for which you think observation or self recording would be appropriate, bearing in mind the reservations. If participatory observation is involved identify whether it would be overt or covert. If the latter, can you justify using it?

Surveys

New information can be obtained through surveys, either by interview or questionnaire. This information may be factual, or concerned with attitudes, or a combination of both.

Interviewing

Interviewing is a system of conducting a survey where people are asked personally for the required information. One disadvantage of this method is that it is very time-consuming. Additionally, because you are employed by a recognised organisation, a health authority or private health care company for example, you will have to decide whether to carry out the interview yourself, and then whether in or out of uniform if you wear one, or whether to use other people to do the interviewing. The aim is to avoid biased answers, so the most appropriate method may depend on the nature of the questions being asked.

Consistency is very important in interviewing. Each respondent, that is each person being interviewed, should be asked the same questions by the same type of interviewer and the answers should be interpreted in the same way. This means that:

● the type of person interviewing should be the same for all respondents

● some form of written questionnaire should be used as a basis for interviews

● if more than one interviewer is used they should be trained to ask questions and interpret answers in the same way.

Postal questionnaires

Postal questionnaires are sent to the respondents to complete in their own time and then return. This is a lot less time-consuming for the researcher than interviewing. The main disadvantage of this method is that it usually gives a low response rate, although this will depend to some extent on the length, complexity and subject matter of the questionnaire. It may also depend upon the time of year since you won't wish to choose a time when everyone is on holiday.

A postal questionnaire should be sent with a covering letter explaining the purpose of the research, requesting help, and impressing upon respondents the value of their contribution. The letter should also promise confidentiality if applicable and give a reasonable date for return. A stamped addressed envelope should also be included where appropriate.

The problem with a low response rate is that it may allow bias to creep in. If, as a student of health care management, you sent out a questionnaire regarding satisfaction with the work of your salaries or wages department it may be that those who are dissatisfied will be more likely to return their questionnaire. Some ways to reduce or eliminate bias are:

● interview all nonrespondents

● interview an appropriate sample of nonrespondents to check that there is no bias

---

ACTION BOX 4.4

Consider your work or study area and identify a suitable subject for a survey.

Decide whether the type of information required would be factual/ attitudinal/both.

Identify the method of survey as likely to be interview/postal questionnaire.

● attempt to increase the response rate by sending out a reminder and second questionnaire to people who have not responded within a certain time.

This may be as far as you want to travel along the subject of surveys. If you now feel that one of the other methods, abstraction from published statistics, data already collected, or observation, or a combination of them, is best suited to your research you need pursue the subject of surveys no further. If, however, you feel that a survey is a vital part of, or will add greatly to the value of your research, you will find assistance in developing the right questions for your survey in Chapter Seven — 'Obtaining your own data'.

Now you are ready to decide on your particular project, and in the next chapter we shall help you to set down the outline of it.

Chapter summary

In this chapter we have looked at ways of collecting statistics. We have described the collection of data from published statistics and from existing sources within an organisation. To conclude the chapter we have described methods of collecting data, observation, self recording, interviewing and postal survey.

References

Cohen C. and Manion L. (1989). *Research methods in education* 3rd Edition. Routledge, London.

Government Statistics (1990). Her Majesty's Stationery Office, London.

Regional Trends. Annual publication. Her Majesty's Stationery Office, London.

Social Trends. Annual publication. Her Majesty's Stationery Office, London.

Further reading

Bell J. (1987). *Doing your research project*. Open University Press, Milton Keynes. At this stage you might find the first two chapters of this book particularly helpful. The book as a whole is very readable.

Crow R. (1984). Observation. In Cormack D.F.S. *The research process in nursing* Chapter 10. Blackwell Scientific Publications, Oxford.
A particularly useful chapter on the observation of human behaviours.

5
Your Project Proposal

Check list

When you have completed this chapter you should have:

- Formulated your project proposal

- Submitted your proposal to the appropriate person(s) for comments

- Considered the comments and where appropriate incorporated suggestions in an amended proposal

We have now covered enough ground for you to be able to get to grips with your own particular project and to commit your ideas to paper. Actually sitting down and doing this is an important step because it will force you to formulate your ideas clearly.

Essential Features

Your project proposal should:

- Identify and explain the problem(s) you think you are solving

- Outline what you hope to achieve by your investigation

- Detail the method(s) of enquiry you intend to use

Considering Constraints

In Chapter Two we identified time constraints as a possible problem. Have a look back at your work on Action Boxes 2.2 and 2.3 now and consider if you think you can complete the project you now have in mind, in the time scales you gave there. For example, if your proposed project involves a large postal survey and you have to have the whole thing completed and submitted in six weeks you will have to think again.

You will also have to consider the availability of other resources such as staff, computing facilities and cash. These constraints will obviously affect the results which can reasonably be expected. If you are going to need other resources make sure that they are available and ask about their use well in advance.

How do you go about obtaining financial support? Good places to start are your line manager, your employing authority and your professional organisation. However, there are a variety of potential sources of funding for research projects and you might find it helpful to read Senga Bond's 'Agencies supportive to nursing research', listed at the end of this chapter which, although directed towards nursing research is applicable to that of other health care professionals.

Now complete Action Box 5·1 (overleaf).

Other Opinions

When the project proposal is written it is important to show it to other people. Whilst it is very gratifying if others congratulate you on proposing a brilliant piece of research, and very painful if they point out an error that's less of a manhole and more of a crater, there are some very sound reasons why you should discuss it with others.

Ethical considerations
If your research involves patients/clients or clinical practice you will have to submit your project proposal to the ethical research committee of your health authority or organisation. Although there is no statutory requirement that there should be Research Ethics Committees in all health districts it is Department of Health policy that health authorities should establish them (Royal College of Physicians 1990).

It is easy to see that undertaking research into the benefits of different treatments may have a direct effect on the people who are subjects of that research. They can be seen as being 'invasive' because they affect the actual physical or psychological care. However, you should also be aware that asking people questions invades their privacy and is therefore a psychological 'intrusion'.

These problems apply whether the people you are researching are well or ill and therefore have ethical implications for you as a student of health care. You

ACTION BOX 5.1

Write out your project proposal in detailed form, including details of timing and your chosen research method. We have included some suggested headings which you may wish to use for the sections of your proposal.

PROJECT PROPOSAL

Name:

Course (if appropriate):

Occupation/professional qualifications/place of work/employer:

Completion date:

Project proposal:

Introduction   (Include reason for choice of subject i.e. problem to be solved)

Aim   (What you hope to achieve by undertaking the research)

Research method   (Use of data in existence, or collection of new data by self recording, observation, interview or postal survey)

Project calender   (A breakdown of how the project will progress by week or month)

Resources required   (Computer access, staff, funding etc. Link to time scale where possible)

could be seriously contravening ethical standards by failing to submit your research proposal for vetting by an ethical committee and could be liable to disciplinary action. It is better to submit a proposal that does not, on consideration, have ethical implications, than omit to submit one that does.

Should people always be told that they are the subjects of research and their consent obtained? The term 'informed consent' is used to describe situations where an individual who is to be the subject of research has all aspects of it explained before consenting to take part. The researcher should bear in mind that patients or staff may at any time withdraw their consent to the study (Wilson-Barnett J. 1984).

If you have any doubts on whether your research proposal should be submitted to your ethical committee, or on the submission procedure to it, the secretary of the committee should be able to advise you.

Professional and managerial support

Obtaining a broad range of opinions is always useful and you will be able to seek the comments of those who have credibility in your eyes and who you feel will be objective without being destructive.

- You may need access to clinical areas to carry out your research and will need to submit your project proposal to appropriate managers to obtain permission for this. Additionally, senior staff can give you further insight into potential ethical problems because of their understanding of the areas they manage.

- If the project is part of a course it will probably be a requirement that you submit your proposal to the course or specialist tutor. Even if it isn't do so anyway to ensure that what you plan to do is appropriate.

- If the work is being done at the request of others, a working party for instance, show them your proposal to make sure that you have correctly interpreted their requirements.

- If the project is in response to a problem you have encountered during your work, show it to others involved. It may be that they see the problem differently.

Who will you submit your project proposal to? Now complete Action Box 5.2 (overleaf).

If this is the first time that someone else has evaluated your work you may well feel a bit discouraged if all their comments seem to be fault finding. Try to hang on to the fact that constructive criticism at this stage will result in an even better project than you had anticipated. If you don't understand their comments, go

---

ACTION BOX 5.2

List the people/committee(s) to whom you will now submit your project proposal, noting for each the reason for their inclusion in the list.

---

back to them and clarify the problems. If you feel really down or discouraged, a good heart to heart talk with your course tutor, a fellow student or colleague can work wonders as a morale booster and put things back into perspective.

Having asked for, and received, comments on your proposal you need to consider them all and revise your proposal if necessary.

ACTION BOX 5.3

Make a summary of comments on your project proposal and decide whether you feel able to pursue your project as initially stated. If you feel that you need to amend the proposal discuss possibilities with your project manager or tutor and note down the amendments decided on.

If a major revision of the project proposal is necessary you should then repeat the tasks in this Action Box by resubmitting your revised proposal for further comment.

If you work for an authority or organisation where a number of people are undertaking research projects at any one time, there may be a central department where project proposals are filed for information. If this is so in your area send them a copy. You will then be ready to plunge into the nitty gritty of your project by starting your literature search, which we describe in the next chapter, and then by undertaking the additional research which you have planned. The final two chapters will then help you with the analysis and presentation of your results.

Chapter summary
In this chapter we have discussed an initial project proposal and the people to whom it might be submitted. We have explored a way of using comments made by them in order to produce an amended project proposal if necessary.

References
Bond S. (1984). Agencies supportive to nursing research. In Cormack D.F.S.

(ed) *The research process in nursing* Chapter 3. Blackwell Scientific Publications, Oxford.

Royal College of Physicians of London (1990). *Guidelines on the practice of ethics committees in medical research involving human subjects* 2nd Edn., Royal College of Physicians, London.

Wilson-Barnett J. (1984). Gaining access to the research site. In Cormack D.F.S. (ed) *Op. cit.* Chapter 8.

Further reading
Bond S. (1984) *See* above.
A useful general chapter.

Wilson-Barnett J. (1984). *See* above.
Although directed at nurses, this chapter is equally relevant to other health care students.

6
Searching the Literature

Check list

When you have completed this chapter you should have:

● Located libraries able to give you reference and/or loan facilities

● Identified other appropriate sources of information

● Identified and located individual books, articles and other items useful to your project literature search.

All projects should involve an examination of existing information on the subject being investigated. In some cases carrying out a full search of all available literature on your subject may be the sole purpose of the project. An example here may be if a committee of which you are a member requires information on setting measurable performance standards before starting work on producing similar sorts of standards for their own health care employees. Equally, though, a thorough search of available literature is an essential stage in any research project, including those specifically designed to produce new data.

Why Search?

Why should you start your search for new data by unearthing all that has gone before on the subject? There are a number of very good reasons. Firstly, a literature search is essential so that you can start your research with as full and deep an understanding of your subject as possible. It may also be necessary to take your research back over a number of years. This means following up every reference which is relevant to the subject of your study whether the material is immediately to hand or not. This may include journals, periodicals, government publications, newspapers and even historical documents in archives and on microfilm. It depends upon the subject and terms of reference.

A literature search will also ensure that you clarify the use of terms, and that where particular words or terminology may have a range of meanings you can define your own use of terminology and support your arguments for that usage with academic evidence. Such evidence is particularly important where you may have to make a choice, for example if your project is concerned with something like the subject of alcoholism. The task in the next action box may prove the point.

ACTION BOX 6.1

Write down your own definition of the term 'alcoholic'.

Fair enough, that's what it means to you but to others it could have meanings as different as 'blind drunk most of the time' and 'dependent upon alcohol without showing any evidence of it'. Convinced? You would need to carry out an extensive literature search to define and settle upon a usage for your own project. You might decide to abandon the use of a term which obviously means different things to different people and to use an alternative term or phrase such as 'alcohol dependent', though it would still need defining!

That example is confined to clarifying the use of just one word, but there are wider advantages of carrying out a literature search. If your research project is, for example, staff appraisal, you will need to read extensively on the subject before undertaking your own research.

Where did the idea of staff appraisal come from or was it always there? How have other people defined, monitored and evaluated staff appraisal? What modifications have been used and with what results? If you carry out and fully document your literature search, your project will have a sound academic base and you will be able to argue from that base against all comers.

Additionally a literature search may:

● Prevent you from duplicating work

● Help you avoid making mistakes other people have made

● Suggest ideas that you hadn't already thought of

● Provide other people's results with which you can later compare your own, although you will have to make sure that you are actually comparing like with like.

Although undertaking a literature search can sound like a vast task, the actual work involved can be minimised if you set about it in a systematic manner.

Where Do You Search?

Firstly you need to identify places where the information you require can be obtained.

You should use a variety of sources in carrying out your search:

Libraries

Obviously you will use public libraries and they will be able to borrow for you, through interlibrary loan, particular volumes which you know you will need and which they do not have in their lists. You must expect these special requests to take some time to meet so make them as soon as possible. You will additionally find that librarians of university, polytechnic and college libraries will usually welcome your use of their libraries for reference purposes, even though you are not a student of that particular establishment. You will probably not be able to borrow books from them but the use of their facilities for reference can be invaluable. All that is usually needed is a telephone call explaining your reasons for wishing to use the particular library. Each librarian will also be able to tell you if that particular library is well supplied in the area of your search. The librarian will also be able to give you details of back numbers of journals which are held.

Professional specialist libraries such as that of the Royal College of Nursing may send lists of items on your subject and copies can then be requested. However, a day actually spent in such a library will greatly speed and assist your search. The library of the King's Fund Centre for Health Services Development is particularly useful for those researching management of institutional or community based health care. The library or resource centre of your own organisation may also yield valuable source material. You should carry out a full search.

Other sources

Other departments or groups of a similar nature may be carrying out, or have completed similar projects, and be able to provide you with useful information and statistics. Contact the appropriate person and ask for any relevant information. State clearly what you require, allow time for them to find it and offer a copy of your project report when it is completed, or a precis if you are making this offer to a large number of people. Interested groups and organisations in your professional speciality can be a valuable source of information as can groups dedicated to people with a particular condition such as the Spastics Society or the Psoriasis Association. Above all you need to think and enquire broadly.

Now, how can you apply that to your particular area of research? Consider your research needs and then plan and make your contacts.

ACTION BOX 6.2

*Tick as appropriate

List the libraries and/or departments and organisations where you plan to start your research and/or note the facilities they offer. We have suggested some useful headings to turn into columns in your file:

| Establishment | *Loan facilities | *Reference facilities | *Request for information |

Searching

The simplest way to approach the task in any library is to go prepared with a list of 'key' words which relate to your particular project subject. You can then search the library subject index using each of the key words in turn. For instance, if you are researching 'food additives', you should start by looking under **food** and then try to find a subsection food **additives**. You may also find it helpful to search under the subheadings of food **allergies**, food **preparation**, food **colourings**, food **flavourings**, or food **preservatives**, and any others you can think of! A book subject index will usually have a logical way of classifying items and may be presented to you either as a card index, on microfiche or on computer.

The card index is simply a set of cards arranged in a number of groupings such as authors, main subjects with subdivisions, and titles. Thus the authors' index will start from Abrahams A., through Abrahams B. and so on. Each card will have the details of one publication by that person on it with a code to tell you under what classification you will find it on the shelf in that library. If you look at the subject index part of the index you will find main subject headings such as 'ethics' with subheadings 'management ethics', 'medical ethics', 'nursing ethics' and so on. The titles index will list, in alphabetical order, the titles of all volumes held.

Alternatively the same indexes may be presented to you on microfiche. These are sheets of acetate which contain, in miniaturised form, details that would take up many individual cards. They are placed on a viewer for scanning.

Some libraries have their indexes on computers so that you can sit at a terminal and bring different details from the indexes onto the screen. Different computers have different systems for use so you need to follow the instructions given in each library.

If you are not familiar with the use of card indexes, microfiche or computer terminals don't hesitate about asking a librarian for help. In our experience librarians are one of the most helpful and patient groups in society! Having said that, once you have asked for help you should learn from it so that you become used to using libraries effectively and independently as rapidly as possible.

When you have a list of likely titles, with their catalogue numbers to help you locate them on the shelves, go off and look at the actual volumes. A quick search of each book's contents list and index can be a useful guide as to how much it can contribute to your studies.

Journal articles are a valuable source of up-to-date information and discussion. Most professional journals and magazines produce a quarterly or annual contents index which should be filed with the year's back copies. Alternatively, some journals publish 'abstracts' which include a short summary of the contents of each article, a great help in deciding whether it is worth while reading the whole item.

'On–line searching'

Obviously you will not be able to search all the libraries in your own country, let alone libraries all over the world. However, articles in journals of your professional discipline or concerned with your particular subject, and held in other libraries or published elsewhere, may be of great value. This is where you may need to use what are called 'on-line' literature searches which contain information on literature on a particular subject held in a variety of locations.

You will need the practical assistance of a librarian for this type of searching. You still need a list of 'key words' from which to start your search just as you do when searching the indexes of one library. The librarian is able to key into information systems in the computers of other libraries and organisations and provide you with a printed list of relevant literature which you can then follow up. Examples of such broad computerised databases are 'Medline' and the Department of Health Database both of which include details of literature on a range of health care subjects. It can be quite expensive to use these resources and the librarian will be able to advise you which databases are likely to provide you with the information you require and how much each search will cost you.

As you make your initial survey of useful material in each library, department or database you may well find that items fall into one of three groups, those obviously essential to the project, those probably useful, and those possibly vaguely useful. When visiting a library to pursue your literature search go armed with this guide and complete the next Action Box task as you do so. You will need three pages in your file, one for each degree of usefulness. List each interesting item on the appropriate page. For a book you will need to note the name of the author, the date of publication, the title, place of publication and the name of the publisher. For an article in a journal, note down the name of the author, the title of the article, the name of the journal, year of publication, the volume number and issue number and the pages on which the article appeared. You will need these details for those volumes to which you refer in your report, and which you will therefore list under the heading 'References'. If any particular page in a book has caught your eye note down the page number and the reason. This will save endless trouble in weeks to come, trying to remember which library and which book or journal a particular table of statistics, that you now realise you desperately need was in.

Be careful that you do not slip into plagiarism: using other peoples' work either 'as is' or in rewritten form, without acknowledging the source. You should also bear in mind that whilst using references to appropriate material is correct the inclusion of large chunks of text that is not your own, however openly acknowledged, is not on!

Now, get to grips with your literature search by completing Action Box 6·3 (overleaf).

Do bear in mind that if you find a reference to a particular set of statistics or item you should trace the original source to check accuracy. Once you have done that your literature search is complete and a fair proportion of the hard work of your project will be over.

In Chapter 4 we also mentioned obtaining data already available in your own organisation. Do not forget this other important source of existing information as it should form part of your literature search.

Chapter summary
In this chapter we have discussed possible sources for a literature search. We have described a systematic way of undertaking a search and of recording details of useful items.

Further reading
Bell J. (1987). *Doing your research project*. Open University Press, Milton Keynes. If you feel that you need more informatiom on literature search Chapter 3 'Reviewing the literature', should help.

ACTION BOX 6.3

Prepare your file sheets using the headings shown here and then start your search!

Sheet 1:

Literature essential to project

Library/ cat.num/ database	Author	Date	Title and comments	Place	Publisher

Sheet 2:

Literature probably useful to project

Library/ cat.num/ database	Author	Date	Title and comments	Place	Publisher

Sheet 3:

Possibly vaguely useful in project

Library/ cat.num database	Author	Date	Title and comments	Place	Publisher

ACTION BOX 6.4

List the data from your own organisation which you intend to use in this project, and which you considered in Chapter 4.

7
Obtaining Your Own Data

Check list

When you have completed this chapter you should have:

● Developed a method of obtaining your own data

● Obtained the data you require

In Action Box 5.1 you identified, in your project proposal, the enquiry method(s) which you proposed to use, and we pointed out earlier that a literature search may well be all that your particular project requires of you. If so, you are lucky, and you can progress straight on to Chapter 8. However, if your project requires other methods of enquiry this chapter will help you to come to grips with, and use, your chosen method or methods.

ACTION BOX 7.1

List the data which your literature search has revealed exists. Decide whether this is adequate or not.

If the data which you have obtained is inadequate for your needs you must decide if the data is in existence somewhere and you just haven't unearthed it yet, or if you will have to produce it yourself. If the former applies, go away and start digging.

If you have now got to set about producing your own data you will need to start by identifying exactly what data you need.

In Chapter 4 we identified three sources of new information:

● observation

● self recording

● survey

and we looked at each so that you could evaluate its use generally and for your own project. Now is the time to develop the materials for, your chosen method, the observation forms, questionnaires and so on, and put them into use.

The remainder of this chapter is in two parts:

Part A — Observation and self recording

Part B — Survey

Work your way through the part or parts which will help you to develop and use the enquiry method identified in your project proposal.

Part A — Observation and Self Recording

Choice of method

If you chose observation or self recording as your method of investigation you now have to plan the details of how you are going to have the information recorded.

As mentioned in Chapter 4 these two methods are very similar. The main difference is that with self recording the people doing the job are collecting the information rather than you or your observers. When choosing between these two methods you should consider the following points:

● **Time available.**   Do you have the time available, or the people, to do observation work? Is it realistic to expect the people doing the job to also record the information? If they are very busy they may not be able to record the data accurately and this would make your results meaningless.

● **Type of information.**   Is it feasible to ask them to record the information you require? For example, they may be able to count how many telephone calls they get but timing them would be more difficult.

● **Vested interests.**   Can you trust the people involved to self record the data accurately or do they have a vested interest in the results of your research?

You need not stick to one of the two methods, you can record some data by self recording and some by observation. If you have doubts about how accurate the self recording is you could do some observation and then compare the results.

Have a brief recap now of the time scales which you detailed in your project proposal in Exercise 5.1, and complete the next Action Box.

ACTION BOX 7A.1

List

● the information to be collected

● the method of collection:
  observation/self recording/combination

● persons carrying out observations/self recording:

To allow time for analysis and reporting of results set yourself a date by which all recording must be completed and note exactly how many days/weeks that gives you.

Designing a form

You will probably need to design your own form for the purpose. Remember that it needs to be set out so that it is clear and easy to use and does not allow any errors through careless recording, for example ticking the '100' column instead of the '10'. Such errors can have unforeseen and far reaching consequences.

ACTION BOX 7A.2

Have a go at designing your form now.

Take your prototype form and discuss it with the people who do the job which is to be observed. If you are using the self recording method these will also be your data collectors. They will be able to give you advice on:

● Whether or not your form covers all regular occurrences

● What problems may arise

● The number of observations likely to be recorded during your planned recording period

● Whether the planned recording period is representative of the rest of the year

If you are using self recording make sure that you have consulted line managers if necessary. It may also be appropriate to arrange a date when you will report back to the people involved, on your results, conclusions and recommendations.

If you are using observers also consult them at this point about the design of your form. At this stage you will also need to consider whether you are going to analyse your results manually or by computer. This may affect the amount of data you want to collect and the design of your recording form so it would be a good idea to seek the advice of a statistics/computing person at this stage. Bear all comments made in the spirit in which they are meant and amend your form accordingly.

Piloting the form

The next stage in the process is to 'pilot' your recording form; this entails running a smaller version of the complete data recording exercise you are planning. Your pilot study need not be large but should be long enough to enable you to identify problems now so that you can solve them before the full data collection exercise begins. When you have completed the pilot study you should be in a position to:

● Speak to the people involved and get their opinions on the accuracy of the data collected and the suitability of the form

● Look at the amount and quality of data collected and confirm that it will satisfy your information requirements and that you will be able to analyse it in the way you intend.

If you have more than one data recorder, piloting the recording form also gives you the opportunity to check that they are recording the same type of information in the same manner.

Run your pilot study and when it is completed identify the items requiring revision.

ACTION BOX 7A.3

Decide how you intend to amend your recording.

Make any changes necessary to your form until you are happy that you have a clear, unambiguous, easily usable form which will allow those recording for you to note without error the data you require. File a copy for future reference and in case anyone loses the master copy for you! Having done that, brief your recorders and start the research.

This is the end of Chapter 7, Part A. If you do not need to design a survey join us again at the end of the chapter for the summary.

Part B — Designing a Survey

This stage will only apply if your project involves using interviews or questionnaires to collect new data. The first task is to decide which questions to include and in what order. The second is to decide who you are going to question.

Choice of questions
When writing these examples of the sort of questions you might set we have used as many different work settings as we possibly could, to shed as much light for you as possible. Usually, of course, all the questions in one survey will relate to one topic!

Open or closed?
The first choice is whether questions should be 'open' or 'closed'. Where questions are open the respondent gives an opinion with no structure. These are time-consuming for interviewers and can cause problems as they are difficult to analyse. Where questions are closed the respondent has a choice of answers

which enables easy analysis. Examples of each type of question are:

open —   what do you think of the present support staff training policy?

closed —   do you think that the amount of time currently spent on support staff training is:

	Tick
too much	☐
about right	☐
too little	☐
don't know	☐

However, although closed questions make analysis easier, it is a good idea to have at least one general comment question at the end of the questionnaire/interview, and perhaps some room for comment after questions which may be difficult to categorise. It can be frustrating for people if they want to say something that you haven't included as one of your alternative answers.

Choose a single answer from a short list of alternatives
These questions can vary considerably as the following examples show:

Have you ever said you were ill when you simply couldn't face going to work?	YES NO
Do you think women are discriminated against in this department?	YES NO UNSURE

How long was it (in minutes) before all the crash team arrived?

	Tick
1 — 5	☐
6 — 10	☐
11 — 15	☐
over 15 mins.	☐

(There is a tendency with this type of question to put 5 — 10, 10 — 15, 15 — 20, etc. However, this is wrong as 10 minutes and 15 minutes would be in two groups.)

		Tick
What is your current grade?	Chiropody student	☐
	Chiropodist	☐
	Senior chiropodist	☐

Numeric rating scale

The respondent ticks one box on the scale:

			Tick
What do you think working in the outpatients department would be like?	Interesting	1	☐
		2	☐
		3	☐
		4	☐
	Boring	5	☐

Several different scales could be applied to the same question. For example the above question could also have an easy/difficult scale. An important point about this type of question is that the terms at each end of the scale should be true opposites.

Verbal rating scales

Similar to numeric rating scales but with a label to each box:

		Tick
How do you rate the job being done by the health visitors in your area?	Very good	☐
	Good	☐
	Average	☐
	Bad	☐
	Very bad	☐

It is important to check that these scales are symmetrical in that there are the same number of terms on either side of the 'average' and that the terms are equivalent, e.g. is 'quite good' equivalent to 'fairly bad'?

Ranking

These request the respondent to rank a list in order of importance.

Please rank the following in order of importance when considering contraceptive advice (1=most important, 4=least important):

Immediate appointment	
Cost	
Staff helpfulness	
Confidentiality	

Select statements from a list

One or more may be selected.

Tick those of the following attributes which you think are important when recruiting occupational therapy students:

	Tick
Educational qualifications	
Written communication skills	
Verbal communication skills	
Physical fitness	
Previous work experience	
Smart appearance	
Compassionate attitude	

Sometimes a limit is put on the number you can select, e.g. you may tick up to three statements. In some cases you could not sensibly pick them all as some would be contradictory.

Where you want to include statements of opinion in your closed questions it is a good idea to have a brainstorming session, preferably with people of the respondent type, in order to get ideas. The aim is to cover most options in your closed questions or you could end up with a lot of 'other' responses or blank boxes.

ACTION BOX 7B.1

Get a group of people together for a brainstorming session. Note down who formed the group and the ideas that were suggested.

Rules for writing questions

Whether questions are open or closed there are five main rules to remember when designing them:

● They must be simple

● They must be written in language the respondent can understand

● They must be unambiguous. An example of an ambiguous question is:

Did you feel better or worse	YES
after the medical social worker called?	NO

● They should not be irrelevant or too personal

● Leading questions should not be asked. An example of a leading question is:

Don't you agree that male physiotherapists are more sympathetic towards women than female physiotherapists?

This suggests that the answer is YES!

Rules for compiling questionnaires

Your questionnaire can be a mixture of different types of open and closed questions, however, there are three main rules to remember:

● It should be as short as possible

● The answers should fall into a logical sequence. Also, excessive use of 'if the answer to 3(c) is 'yes' go to 5(d)' type questions should be avoided. They can lead to omissions and confusion.

● It must yield results in a form suitable for the analysis intended.

Now have a go at putting all that into practice. Remember the advice given and check as you go along that you are heeding it, particularly in relation to **simplicity, unambiguity and relevance.**

ACTION BOX 7B.2

Design your prototype questionnaire.

Testing the questionnaire

When you have drawn up your questionnaire the next stage is to get other people's opinion of it. If possible include people with survey experience in addition to those with knowledge of the questionnaire subject matter. Also, if you plan to have the data resulting from your survey computerised by someone else it is essential that they see the prototype. Whether or not computerisation is warranted will depend on the number of respondents, the number and type of questions and the complexity of the analysis you are hoping to do.

When giving your questionnaire to anyone for comment ensure that they have a clear idea of what you are trying to achieve as otherwise they will not be able to judge the relevance of your questions.

ACTION BOX 7B.3

When you have received all the comments put them together by placing them in similar groups such as those recommending that a particular question is clarified or that you have more questions on a particular subject.

Consider the main groups of comments and amend your questionnaire accordingly.

Identifying the respondents

Once you have made any changes resulting from people's comments the next step is to identify the group of people for whom your survey is intended.

There are three problems to consider when identifying this group:

● what type of people

● how many people

● how to select the individuals.

The group of people from whom you want to collect information is called the 'survey population' and it is very important to define this properly before you send out questionnaires or start interviewing. For example, if you are collecting information on health centre receptionists, is the survey population all health centre staff or just health centre receptionists? This depends on whether you want to collect information from receptionists on their job or if you want to know how a cross-section of staff see the receptionists' role.

If the whole survey population is small and easily surveyed it may be possible to examine every member of it. However, if the survey population is large it may only be possible to examine part of it, a sample. Thus, if the population was receptionists it might be possible to survey them all, whereas if it was all health centre staff it might be necessary to take a sample.

Whether or not all the population is surveyed and the size of the sample will be determined by:

● **Available time.**
This affects interviews more than postal questionnaires as they are very time-consuming. As well as the time to conduct the interview time will also have to be allowed for interviewer training and travelling.

● **Available money.**
Printing, postage and time spent interviewing all cost money. When deciding on the sample size it is necessary to consider the value of the resulting information, e.g. is it going to form the basis of a major policy decision for your organisation or form a small part of a course you are taking.

● **Statistical accuracy required.**
We cannot assume that the results we get from our sample will be the same as would be obtained if all the population were surveyed. However, the more responses the results are based on, the nearer the two will be.

● **Response rate.**

If you are expecting a response rate of less than 100% build this into your sample size. For example, if you want 200 respondents and you expect a 70% response rate divide 200 by 70 and multiply the result by 100 to get an adjusted sample size (286). Do not just send out 200 and hope for the best. It is difficult to predict response rates but it is reasonable to suppose that certain topics and populations will give higher response rates than others. The pilot survey will also give you an idea of the response rate you can expect. You should not forget that however many questionnaires you send out a low response rate may itself cause bias in your results.

The relative importance of the points mentioned above will depend on the type of questions you are asking and the purpose of your survey. If you need greater details on the subject of sample sizes you should refer to the text by Gregory and Ward listed in the further reading section of this chapter.

Once the nature of the population and the size of the sample have been decided it is necessary to find a list of people of the chosen population. This will of course vary according to the nature of your project, however, three commonly used sources are:

● list of employees of appropriate grade or occupation, from personnel departments. You may need to approach both your own department and those in other health authorities or health care organisations.

● electoral register. This can be used when surveying the public. Copies are available at council offices and in public libraries in the chosen location.

● public relations or similar departments. These can be used when surveying members of the public who have had recent contact with your organisation.

Piloting the questionnaire

Now that you have a list of your intended population select a group to include in a pilot study. Keep a note of those whom you select so that you can avoid reusing them for your actual survey. It is difficult to give a definitive answer on how big a pilot survey should be. However, it should be large enough for you to identify problems **before** the full data collection exercise is underway.

Now complete Action Box 7B·4.

Your pilot survey will tell you how long it takes to deliver an interview questionnaire and highlight any difficulties for the interviewer. It is a good idea to add a final question for the respondent to comment on the questionnaire itself so that any difficulties encountered can be described. On postal questionnaires

---

ACTION BOX 7B.4

Identify the group of people who are to be your survey population and the source from which you will obtain their details.

List the names/addresses/departments and/or health authority or other organisation if appropriate, of those who you hope will take part in your pilot study.

---

respondent difficulties may additionally be identified by missed questions and comments written next to questions where a closed response was requested.

It is also a good idea to look at the pilot survey results with a view to analysis and check if the questions are set out in the best way to give the results in the form you want. Now, pilot!

When your pilot study is completed identify items which require revision.

ACTION BOX 7B.5

List the items that require revision and describe, for each one, the specific problem and how you intend to overcome it.

Now produce the final draft of your questionnaire.

Sampling
The next step is to select the required number for your survey from the population list. Three commonly used methods of selection are described below:

Random sampling
Each member of the population is numbered and then random sample number tables are used to select the required sample size. Random number tables will usually include instructions for their use and can be found in books of statistical tables such as that by Murdoch and Barnes listed in the further reading list. Alternatively, basic statistical textbooks often include some statistical tables in appendices.

Systematic sampling

This is a short cut method for obtaining a virtually random sample. If a 10% sample was required then it could be selected by taking every tenth item in the population, providing that there is no regularity within the population such that items ten spaces apart have some special quality. For example, every tenth house number may be on the same side of the street and this may matter if there are different types of housing on different sides of the street. Given that proviso this method is acceptable for the majority of research projects.

Stratified sampling

This method reduces sampling error as it makes the sample match the population in some important aspect(s) thus making it more representative. For instance, if surveying patients cared for in 'mixed male and female' wards, then if 40% of these had been male you may want 40% of your sample to be male. Once you have split the population into groups you can sample from within each of these groups using either random or systematic sampling.

When selecting a sample for an interview survey it is a good idea to select some people for a reserve list. Then, if it is not possible to contact a particular member of your sample, one from the reserve list can be substituted. However, before you make a substitution think carefully about why you cannot contact the person originally selected. For example, if you are interviewing on a weekday afternoon it may be that all those you are able to contact do not work, whereas those you are missing do. If you then substitute those you cannot get hold of with non-working people, you will have a biased sample. Also, you should not reuse

---

ACTION BOX 7B.6

Record the details of your postal or interview survey, using the headings:

Population.

Proportion of the population, identifying whether you are using all the population or a sample.

If you are using a sample, whether it is random, systematic or stratified.

List those selected to be your respondents noting their name, address, department and health authority or organisation if appropriate.

Now, send out your questionnaires or set your interviewers to work.

---

individuals who took part in your pilot study, so cross check for this and substitute a matching 'reserve' if this has happened.

Remember to keep accurate notes of those surveyed, recording details of all interviews undertaken and questionnaires sent out and returned. Always record these items at once and file safely. If you do not, you may find that several days and many questionnaires later, terminal confusion sets in!

Chapter summary

In this chapter we have described the collection of new data by observation, self recording and survey. We have then explained the questionnaire process in detail.

Further reading

Belson W.A. (1981). *The design and understanding of survey questionnaires.* Gower, Aldershot.
Provides a sound base for the development of questionnaires.

Clegg F. (1982). *Simple statistics.* Cambridge University Press, Cambridge.
Approaches the more complex uses of statistical evidence in a relatively simple way.

Gregory D. and Ward H. (1978). *Statistics for business.* McGraw-Hill, London.
This book has useful chapters covering the collection of data (Chapter 2) and sampling and sample size (Chapters 12 and 14).

Huff D. (1973). *How to lie with statistics.* Penguin Books, London.
It may be hard to imagine a 'couldn't put it down' book about statistics but this is it! Use it as a check on your own statistics before you commit your results to your research report.

Murdoch J. and Barnes J.A. (1986). *Statistical tables for science, engineering, management and business studies.* Macmillan, London.
As mentioned, this includes random number tables.

Oppenheim A.N. (1985). *Questionnaire design and attitude measurement.* Gower, Aldershot.
Another good text on questionnaire development.

8
Analysing Your Data

Check list

When you have completed this chapter you should have:

- Analysed your research results

- Written, submitted and/or circulated your report

A variety of methods of analysing data are discussed below, these range from totals and percentages to more complicated statistical analysis. What is appropriate will depend on the nature of the data you have collected and also your level of experience in such techniques. All of the methods described below are covered in more detail in the text books listed in the further reading section at the end of the chapter. However, if you are still unsure after reading these then find a suitably experienced person to help you.

Graphics, that is the diagrammatic representation of statistics, also play a major part in the analysis and presentation of results and these will be discussed in the second half of this chapter.

The first step is to list all the data you have obtained, you can then bear it in mind as you read this chapter.

ACTION BOX 8.1

List all the data which you have obtained and want to analyse and include in your report.

Analysis of Results

Response Rates

If you are analysing survey results you will need to include a response rate in your report. For a postal survey this would simply be the number of questionnaires returned as a percentage of the number sent out. For an interview survey it would be the number of interviews conducted as a percentage of the sample size i.e. the actual divided by the expected multiplied by 100. For example, if we sent out 75 questionnaires but only received 53 back the response rate would be:

$$(53/75) \times 100 = 70.666667\%$$

It is normal to give such results to the nearest whole number or to one decimal place. If a figure is 5 or more it should be rounded up, otherwise it should be rounded down. The above result would be:

70.7% to one decimal place
71% to the nearest whole number

If the response rate was 70.321412% the result would be:–

70.3% to one decimal place
70% to the nearest whole number

ACTION BOX 8.2

If you are analysing survey results calculate your response rate.

If you have any information on non-respondents you may want to include this in your report.

For example, lets say that 25% of our clients come from area A and 75% from area B. We sent out 200 questionnaires, 50 to clients in area A (25%) and 150 to clients in area B (75%). We received 150 back which is a response rate of 75% ($150/200 \times 100$). However, if this is made up of 10 from area A ($10/50 \times 100 = 20\%$ response rate) and 140 from area B ($140/150 \times 100 = 93\%$ response rate) we should mention this in our report. Although our sample represented the proportion of clients in each area our returned questionnaires do not.

If the response rate is low there should be some discussion included on the possible reasons for this and the implications for the usefulness of the results.

ACTION BOX 8.3

Note down any information you have on the non-respondents.

Grouping Data

Before you can analyse your data it will need to be in a suitable form. In some cases this is easy. If we asked hospital switchboard operators to rate their job on an interesting/boring scale of 1(interesting) to 5(boring) the answers would be 1, 2, 3, 4 or 5. However, in some cases there is a much wider range of possible figures. If we collected information on how long the switchboard operators have been employed in their current posts we might have many different values which would need summarising before we could analyse them.

We need to identify the highest and lowest values and subtract one from the other to obtain the range. The number and size of groupings can then be decided. This number of groupings is usually around 5-10 and should be chosen to give equal class sizes with logical break points between them. If you have too few classes you are losing detail if you have too many you are defeating the point of summarising the data.

If the highest length of service for the switchboard operators was 11 years and the lowest was 2 weeks the following grouping would be suitable:

under 2 years
2   and under   4 years
4   and under   6 years
6   and under   8 years
8   and under 10 years
10 and under 12 years

There should be a group for every figure and no figure should fit into more than one group. For these reasons both of the following examples would be wrong.

0 to 2 years
2 to 4 years
4 to 6 years...

This is wrong as two years would fit into both the first and second group.

0 to 2 years
3 to 5 years
6 to 8 years...

This is wrong as two years six months would not fit into any of the groups, it would fall between the first and second.

Once you have calculated your response rate and grouped any data where necessary, you need to consider which types of analysis will be the most appropriate. We will discuss them generally now before, in you work on your own data (Action Box 8.4).

Counts, Total and Percentages

The following steps apply equally to grouped or ungrouped data.

● Count how many responses/figures go into each category. The number in each group is known as the frequency.

● Total these figures and check that they add to the expected number. If they do not due to missing responses you will need to decide what to do, this will be discussed after the example below.

● Calculate percentages for each category by dividing the number in that category by the total and multiplying it by 100, for example $(6/53) \times 100 = 11.32075$. To one decimal place this would be 11.3%, to the nearest whole number 11%.

● Check that the percentages add to 100% although there may be a slight error (0.1% if using one decimal place, 1% if using whole numbers etc.) due to rounding.

The example below shows the results for a survey question with 53 respondents:

Do you find the job of switchboard operator?

			Freq.	%
Fasy	1	=	6	11%
	2	=	14	26%
	3	=	16	30%
	4	=	12	23%
Difficult	5	=	5	9%
			53	100%

The above percentages add to 99 not 100 due to rounding errors but 100% has been written as 53 is 100% of 53.

If your numbers do not add to the expected total for a particular question you will need to decide what to do. Firstly, don't try and guess what the missing respondent meant, just leave them out. Secondly, have a look at the whole questionnaire, if it has a lot of spoiled questions it may be better to add it to the nonrespondents and omit it from the analysis completely i.e. reduce the response rate to 52 of 75 and analyse all the questions for those 52 respondents.

If there are no problems with the rest of the questionnaire you can analyse the particular question for 52 respondents and the rest for 53. This could be done by saying either '52 of the 53 respondents answered this questions as follows' and then give the figures adding to 52 or by including the missing item as an additional category as follows:

			Freq.	%
Easy	1	=	6	11%
	2	=	14	26%
	3	=	16	30%
	4	=	12	23%
Difficult	5	=	4	8%
Missing		=	1	2%
			53	100%

Means and Modes

These commonly used statistics are the average (mean) and the most common value (mode).

The mean for the above switchboard operator example would be calculated by multiplying each of 1 to 5 by their frequency, totalling these figures and then dividing the result by the number of respondents.

	Value	Freq.	No × Value
Easy	1	6	6
	2	14	28
	3	16	48
	4	12	48
Difficult	5	5	25
		53	115

Mean Rating = 115/53 = 2.9

When you have calculated the mean look at your figures again and check that the mean looks sensible given the range of results.

The mode is simply the most common value, in this case 3 which has a frequency of 16.

These two statistics have to be calculated slightly differently for grouped data. To obtain the mean we first of all find the midpoint for each group and then do the calculation using this value.

For example the number of patients attending 100 outpatient clinic sessions:

Patients Attending	Freq.	Midpoint	Midpoint × Freq.
16–20	19	18	342
21–25	29	23	667
26–30	18	28	504
31–35	15	33	495
36–40	11	38	418
41–45	8	43	344
	100		2770

Mean = 2770/100 = 27.7 patients attending

The modal group would be the group with the highest frequency.

Measures of Dispersion

The mean is a useful statistic but it does not tell the whole story. For example both of the following sets of results have means of 2.9 but if you look at the percentages there is a different pattern in the results.

		GROUP 1		GROUP 2	
		Freq.	%	Freq.	%
Easy	1	5	11%	16	30%
	2	14	26%	22	40%
	3	16	30%	9	17%
	4	12	23%	5	9%
Difficult	5	5	9%	2	4%
		53	100%	53	100%

Therefore in addition to the mean and mode it is useful to give some value to the spread or 'dispersion' of the information. This could be done by:

● Providing the percentage share for each value as above.

● Providing the information in graphical form e.g. a pie or bar chart. These will be explained in the second part of this chapter.

● Calculating the range, this is the highest minus the lowest value. However, this value does not always illustrate the differences in two sets of figures, for example it is 4 for both the examples above, and it can also be affected by extreme values.

● Calculating statistics such as the mean deviation or standard deviation. Information on how to calculate these can be found in the books listed as further reading at the end of the chapter.

Cross Tabulations

You may want to link certain items of information from your questionnaire to each other. For example, length of service and how easy/difficult people find the job. If so, you will need to draw up a matrix as below and count how many go into each square.

	Easy 1	2	3	4	Difficult 5	Total
less than 2 years						
2 – less than 4 years						
4 – less than 6 years						
6 – less than 8 years						
8 – less than 10 years						
10 – less than 12 years						
Total						

There is a test known as a Chi-squared test which measures the significance of the patterns which are illustrated by such tables. This test, and the others covered below, are described in the books listed in the further reading section at the end of the chapter.

Comparisons

You may have surveyed two groups, or split your respondents into two groups, and want to compare the results. For example we might have surveyed the public in two areas asking – How do you rate the job being done by the health visitors in your area?

		AREA A		AREA B	
(1)	Very Good	3	5%	2	4%
(2)	Good	21	38%	10	21%
(3)	Average	25	45%	20	42%
(4)	Bad	5	9%	11	23%
(5)	Very Bad	1	2%	5	10%
		55	100%	48	100%
Mode		3 = 'Average'		3 = 'Average'	
Mean		2.6		3.1	

We cannot compare numbers as there are different totals in each group. However we can compare the mode and the mean and look at the spread of the responses.

There are tests known as T-tests which enable you to use the sample sizes, the means and standard deviations (mentioned above) to test whether apparent differences are significant, i.e. are the health visitors in Area B perceived to be doing a significantly better job that those in Area A. An important point is do not use the word significant when discussing your results unless you have proved that something is *statistically* significant.

Correlation and Regression

You may want to test whether two factors are related, this is known as correlation. For example, the age of patients and the amount of time it takes them to recover from a particular illness. The first task is to plot each pair of variables on a graph with one variable along the horizontal axis and one along the vertical axis. This is known as a scattergraph and is described in more detail in the second part of the chapter. The points on the graph can then be examined for a pattern, e.g. Does recovery time increase with age?

In addition to looking at the graph there are two calculations you can do. The first, regression analysis, will enable you to draw a straight line through the points on the graph showing the relationship between the two sets of data. The second, correlation, will enable you to calculate a statistic which will tell you how strong the relationship is and you can then look this up in tables to see whether or not it is significant.

It is very important to note that even when two variables are strongly correlated it does not necessarily mean that an increase in one variable is the cause of the increase or decrease in the other. The high correlation may be due to coincidence or to a third factor.

Trends over time

You may have a series of information over time. The first thing that you should always do with information of this type is to plot it on a line graph with time (months, years etc.) on the horizontal axis and the variable on the vertical axes. Seasonal influences in the data may disguise the trend. However, this can calculated using a method known as the moving average. These calculations result in a trend line which can also be plotted in the graph.

Analysing opinions

In this chapter so far we have covered the analysis of numeric data but you may have collected peoples opinions on a subject. There is a danger with this type of information of quoting the statements which support your argument without summarising all of the responses. If the number of comments is not too high they can be listed in an appendix, either in respondent order or grouped by type. If there are a large number then a summary could be included of the number making the same types of comment.

The above are some techniques which may be of use to you. Now decide how to analyse your data.

ACTION BOX 8.4

Look at the list you made for Action Box 8.1. Write next to each how to analyse the data you have collected and then perform the appropriate calculations.

Graphics

In addition to tables of figures you might like to represent your data graphically. The use of appropriate graphs can be very effective, as people tend to find them easier to interpret than tables of figures. Two general points to remember when creating your graphs are:

● Each graph should have a heading, labels on both axes and a key if more than one type of shading has been used. If there can be any doubt as to the exact nature of the data graphed, provide an explanation in a footnote. This point applies equally to figures presented in tabular form.

● If you are going to have to produce more than one copy of your report and do not have access to a colour photocopier then use different styles of shading rather than different colours on your graphs.

There are several different types of graph you could use depending on the nature of your data, and which we will now discuss.

A set of bars of equal width with half-bar spaces between them. Bar charts are usually used to represent the size of different categories. For example the **number** of outpatients in each of four districts.

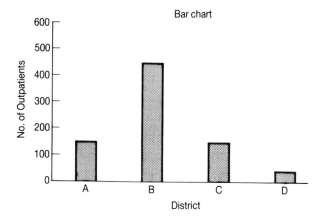

Bar chart

Multiple bar charts can also be produced which have more than one value for each category. For example the number of outpatients in two different periods.

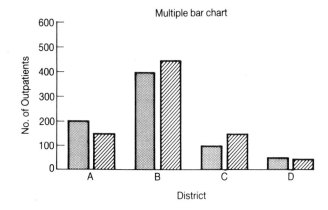

Multiple bar chart

Stacked bar charts show how each category can be broken down in some way. For example, the number of outpatients in period 2 can be broken down into those that were orthopaedic and those that were not. These graphs may become confusing if the bars are divided into more than two or three sections.

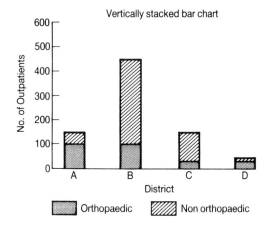

Vertically stacked bar chart

Traditionally bar charts have been drawn horizontally but computer graphics packages, such as the one used to produce the above graphs, tend to print them vertically. The important point is to leave a gap between the bars.

Pictograms are bar charts made up of pictures rather than bars. For example if each 50 outpatients were represented by a stick figure the period 2 district A figure of 150 could be shown by three figures on top of each other instead of a bar.

Cartograms are a way of presenting geographical data. For example to show the death rate in each district of a health authority we could divide it into districts and then show each district according to the death rate. With cartograms it is important to have a key showing what value or range of values each shade represents.

A pie chart is a circle where each segment represents a share of the whole. An example of its use would be to illustrate the proportion (%) of a region's outpatients that were treated in each of the districts. If you want to draw attention to one or more segments, such as **District A** in the example, they can be 'exploded' Instructions on how to construct a pie chart manually are also given in the books listed in the further reading section.

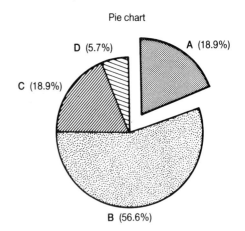

Pie chart

D (5.7%) A (18.9%)

C (18.9%)

B (56.6%)

Histograms look similar to the bar charts we have shown except that there are no gaps between the bars. They are used for continuous or grouped data, e.g. height or weight of children, rather than data in categories e.g. hair colour or employment grade. More information on histograms and their construction can be found in the basic statistical books given in the further reading section at the end of the chapter.

Scatter diagrams are a way of comparing two sets of figures to see how they vary from one another. For example we could compare the number of patients with hospital costs by:

● marking a scale for patients numbers on one axis

● marking a scale for costs on the other axis

● putting a cross on the graph for each pair of figures

We could then look for a trend in the crosses — do costs rise with the number of patients?

Line graphs are useful for showing trends over time. For example, we could have a line showing the total number of outpatients each period for 20 periods. Alternatively there could be 4 lines on the graph, one for each of the districts identified in the previous examples. This might enable us to compare different trends but could be confusing if the lines are very close together or cross over.

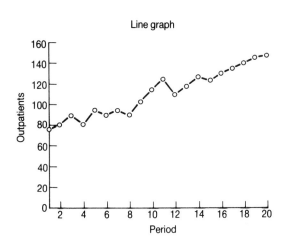

Line graph

ACTION BOX 8.5

List the graphs you need to prepare for your data.

Summary
In this chapter we have described the analysis of research results and the preparation of graphics

Further reading
Gregory D. and Ward H. (1978). *Statistics for business*. McGraw-Hill, London.

Mulholland H. and Jones C.R. 1968 *Fundamentals of statistics*. Butterworth: Heinemann Educational, London.

Rowntree, D. 1981. *Statistics without tears: a primer for non-mathematicians.* Pelican, London.

These all contain sections on preparing tables, the first is particularly good.

9
Reporting Your Results

Check list

When you have completed this final chapter you should have:

- Written, submitted and/or circulated your report

Writing the Report

Word limits
When deciding on the presentation of your report you should consider its length. You may be convinced that only a report three inches thick will do justice to your topic but if those to whom you submit it lack the hours necessary to wade through it you will have wasted your time. If the project is to be submitted as a piece of course work you will probably already have been given a 'word limit'. It is helpful to remember as a rough guide that an A4 sheet of average handwriting contains about 300 words. A typewritten sheet of the same size contains about 250 words if double spaced and 500 words if single spaced. It is usual to present such projects typewritten and double spaced. Appendices and bibliography are usually additional to given word limits.

ACTION BOX 9.1

Identify the number of words you aim to have as a limit for your report, excluding appendices and bibliography.

The format

In writing your report you may find it helpful to follow a structured format that will ensure it conforms to accepted academic principles and also does what you want it to do. The structure we shall guide you through here should be suitable for the majority of project reports. Again, if the project is to be submitted as part of course work you may find that you are expected to use a given format.

Official reports usually have their paragraphs numbered according to the chapter or section number and the relationship of each paragraph to that chapter. Thus paragraph eight in Chapter 1 is 1.8, and paragraph four in Chapter 6 is 6.4. If a chapter has sections this process can be extended so that paragraph three in section five of Chapter 1 is numbered 1.5.3.

References

You will want to make use of the references obtained in your literature search. There are a number of acceptable ways of using these in your text. You may, for example in discussing quality control, refer as follows:

> Discussions on quality assurance often overlook explicit agreement on the values of professional groups and the society or community served. (Kitson A. 1989).

Alternatively you might quote Kitson directly:

Kitson has stated that

> "Explicit agreement on the values of the professional groups, and also on the society or community which it serves, is another area overlooked in discussions on quality assurance." (Kitson 1989).

There are other ways of using references in text, for example putting a number by the reference itself, and the number and relevant details at the bottom of the page, but we feel that the first example given, without using direct quotation, and with details tabulated in a reference list is particulsrly suitable for project reports.

Whatever format you choose in the text the references must be listed, in alphabetical order, in a specific way. This listing should give the author, by surname and initials, the date of publication of the volume, the title of the volume, its place of publication and the name of the publisher. The example we have used would appear in the reference list as:

Kitson A. (1989) *A framework for quality*. Harrow, Scutari Press.

If your reference is from a journal or magazine you should include the title of the article, the title, volume and issue number of the journal, and the pages, using the abbreviation 'p or pp' for 'page or pages', on which the article appeared, for example:

Coyle L. A. & Souop A. G.. Innovation Adoption Behaviour Among Nurses. *Nursing Research.* 1990, **39**, No. 3, pp176–180.

We shall return to these additional details when we reach the bibliography and references page of your report, if that is where you choose to list them.

Sections of the report

There are nine distinct 'parts' which you need to prepare:

the cover

the table of contents

a summary

an introduction and methodology

the results

your conclusions

your recommendations

any appendices

your references and bibliography

Each Action Box in the next series takes you through preparing one of the parts so that when you have completed them you will have completed your report. It will probably be simplest to make rough notes in your file and then write up your report as a whole when you have completed the notes.

The cover

Not always as simple as it sounds! It should usually have not only the title of your project on it but also the date, your name and that of your organisation if appropriate, and any other details you feel are required given the reason for undertaking the project. Remember that the title often sets the tone and influences the way in which readers approach your work. Finalise the wording now, and also the layout you require.

ACTION BOX 9.2

Prepare a full size rough draft of your cover.

Table of contents

The table of contents lists all those items which your report contains. That means that in addition to listing chapters or sections, and possibly their subsections, you must list illustrations and diagrams, references and bibliography, and any appendices.

You may need to return to this Action Box task later to amend it as necessary. If the pages are to be numbered you will definitely have to leave that part of it until the end.

ACTION BOX 9.3

Make a rough draft of your contents page using the headings below

Contents   Page

Summary

Most reports commence with a summary which contains very briefly the main points of the report. You will need to state, virtually in one sentence each, the reason for researching the particular subject, the method chosen, the results, and your conclusions and main recommendations. In fact a summary of all the parts of the report which are going to appear in detail in the main body of it.

ACTION BOX 9.4

Prepare your summary now.

Introduction and methodology

Next you need to write an introduction that describes the reasons for doing the research. Not the 'because it's part of my course' variety, but the 'staff turnover had been rising steadily without any readily identifiable cause' sort!

This part of the report should also describe your methodology by outlining the methods of investigation you used.

ACTION BOX 9.5

Prepare your introduction and methodology sections using those two headings.

The results

This part of the report sets out the findings of the research, discusses them and makes deductions from them. Information which is for reference, such as statistical analysis tables and graphs always appears in appendices being referred to as 'Appendix 1' etc. when discussed in the text. For example:

The number of employees leaving within 12 months of commencing employment with the department was 12%, constituting 0.4% of the total work force (Appendix 1, p68).

You will obviously therefore need to prepare these appendices and file them here now, although we shall put them in their proper place in Activity Box 8.11.

This part of the report should also include an examination of the possible courses of action with an assessment of the implications of each. You should not draw conclusions or make recommendations at this stage.

ACTION BOX 9.6

Prepare your 'Results' section of your report, using that heading, and a second heading 'Possible courses of action'

List appendices to be prepared

Conclusions

You will now need to draw your conclusions based on the evidence and alternatives given in the previous part of the report. No new material should appear in this section.

ACTION BOX 9.7

Prepare the 'Conclusions' part of your report.

Recommendations

From your conclusions you will then evolve your recommendations. State what action you advise on the strength of the evidence, the discussion and the conclusions.

ACTION BOX 9.8

Prepare the 'Recommendations' section of your report.

Appendices

Now make sure that the appendices that you prepared as part of Action Box 8.8 are in order.

ACTION BOX 9.9

Check and number your appendices and their titles.

Don't forget to add these into the contents list that you prepared in Action Box 8.5.

Bibliography and references

This list should include any books or articles directly referred to in the text plus any other books, articles or other references that have been useful. Remember that you need the name of the author, the date of publication of the volume, the title of the volume, its place of publication and the name of the publisher of each volume, plus the title of an individual article, and the title and issue number of the journal in which the article appeared. If you were efficient you included this information for all the items you consulted in your literature search in your work for Action Box 6.3, so the task of selecting those you have used and transferring the details here should not be too difficult.

It may also be appropriate here to include acknowledgement of contribution made by individuals, groups and departments. Not only will you naturally be grateful to them but such acknowledgement may motivate them to participate in future research.

ACTION BOX 9.10

Check your bibliography and references using the following list to ensure that you have all the details needed:

Author   Date   Title/Journal   Place of publication
Publisher and pages

Circulating Your Report

If your project has been undertaken as part of a course you will naturally submit it as specified by the course tutor. Similarly, research generated through working parties will be submitted to the initiators who will, you no doubt hope after all your work, act upon it. As with your research proposal, if your organisation has a central department which monitors in-house research you should provide them with a copy of your report. If you submitted your research proposal to an ethical committee they should also be sent a copy of the report. Remember also those organisations or companies who provided you with information and to whom you promised a copy or precis of your completed project. Now, fulfil your promises and obligations!

ACTION BOX 9.11

List those to whom you will send copies of your report and note when you have done so.

Presenting Your Findings

It may also be appropriate for you to give a presentation of your results to interested parties. For example if you made use of self recording it may be that you agreed to present your findings to those involved, or you may be required to give a presentation as part of related course work. Many of us find giving presentations an ordeal, but if you consider the following points when preparing your presentation it may not be so difficult:

● **Take the level of knowledge** of the audience and the nature of their interest into account.

● **Consider the intended length** of the presentation session. Have a practice run to check that you will be able to fill or fit in with the time scale.

● **Delivery is important!** It is better not to simply read a prepared script out word for word. Try using headings on cards for all the points you want to cover. You can then use them as 'triggers' for what you say, expanding on them as you go and look at your audience more often as you are speaking. Your presentation should thus be more natural.

● **Allow time for questions** and be prepared for any that are likely to be put to you. It is a good idea to ask a friend to read your report and think up the most awkward questions possible so that you can consider how you would answer them before you get to the presentation!

● **Consider the use of equipment** available to you such as a flip chart or overhead projector. If you use an overhead projector some points to bear in mind are:

— slides should not be cluttered; try using lists of 'key' points to expand on verbally

— graphs are usually a better method of presenting data visually than figures

— don't obstruct your audience's view of the screen

— switch off the projector when you are not referring to a slide, otherwise the noise may prove distracting

● **If you are not a natural music hall turn,** don't try to be funny. You may die on your feet and your research may be viewed unfavourably as a result. This last Action Box of the guide helps you to prepare for a 'live' presentation.

ACTION BOX 9.12

Consider the group to whom you are presenting your project. Identify any characteristics of the group that you should bear in mind.

Note the time allowed and write down the headings from which you will develop your 'delivery'.

Consider the questions you think you are likely to be asked.

Finally list the equipment you plan to use and the items such as projector slides you need to prepare.

There now remains only a final summary of the work of this chapter and the guide as a whole.

Final summary
In this chapter we have worked through the process of writing a project report and considered appropriate circulation and presentation of the completed report.

We hope that you have found the guide helpful and that you feel that you have achieved the overall aim, that you have:

Completed a simple research project to your own satisfaction and to that of those requiring you to undertake it.

Good luck with future research projects!
Dianne Owen and Moya Davis.